Laure Goldbright

||||| ||| ||||||||||||| ||| |||||
I0101678

Colon Cleansing and Its Benefits for Health and Skin: A Testimonial

How I regained a flat stomach, slim waist, peaceful sleep, and healthy skin without age spots by colonic irrigation

Buenos Books America

www.buenosbooks.us

First published in French by Buenos Books International, Paris, as *Témoignage sur les Bienfaits de l'Hygiène Intestinale*

ISBN: 978-1-963580-00-6

Imprint

Buenos Books America

www.buenosbooks.us

"Men will come to such a state of abasement that they will be happy that others benefit from their suffering, or the loss of their true wealth, health."

Leonardo da Vinci, The Notebooks

"Nature itself, when we let it be, gently pulls itself out of the mess it has fallen into. It is our worry, it is our impatience that spoils everything, and almost all men die from their remedies, not from their illnesses. "

Molière, The Imaginary Patient

Men will come to such a state of ... sense that they will be happy that others benefit from their sufferings, or the ... some true health."

Leonardo da Vinci, The Notebooks

... till ... then we learn beg, only ... is ... of ... in ... fallen ... to ... one worry, it is one ... that has spoke ... ing and almost all ... ... articles, ... in their illness.

The Humanure Handbook

4

INTRODUCTION

In my forties, while having been fortunate enough to be in near perfect health until then, I started suffering from intense bloating. The crisis started around three in the morning, and soon my stomach was sore and as big as that of a woman in late pregnancy. The bloating crisis lasted a few hours, during which time I evacuated the gas in both directions using self-massage, finally falling asleep in the early hours of the morning, just a few hours before getting up to go to work.

There is no need to tell you how exhausted I was, not to mention the horrible recurring nightmares full of violent and bloody scenes caused by these disturbances in my digestive tract. The horror movies served up by TV and the cinema have nothing on those I created for myself in my sleep. At the time, I also had another recurring dream theme that I will discuss later in the conclusion of this book, because this theme, according to my research, is very common in people with congested bowels. Long before we get sick, thanks to our dreams, we have an extra chance to avoid sickness through subconsciously understanding that something is wrong with the body and taking immediate action to remedy it.

When my health issues started, I couldn't understand what was happening to me. Why was I having these bouts of aerophagia? How could it be that my belly would start to swell so much every night around three o'clock, no matter what I had eaten and even if I had skipped dinner? I decided to consult a doctor, who told me with a smile that my problems were not serious, that they were simply due to gastric acidity, and that a commonly prescribed antacid would solve them very easily. So he prescribed me the usual miracle drug for patients with stomach acidity. The doctor didn't try to understand why at this time in my life my body had become imbalanced and he gave me no information on what I could do to regain this lost balance. I was visibly bothering him with all the questions he couldn't answer.

For me, these attacks of aerophagia were serious because they deeply disturbed my sleep. I knew full well that if I took this medication long-term to relieve my symptoms and continued ignoring my body's cry for help, it would lead to serious and possibly incurable illness in the future. I also realized that I was not the only one suffering from this problem. Aerophagia and disturbances in the digestive tract are common and people survive them with the help of laxatives, antacids, etc. Pharmaceutical companies make a lot of money on remedies that , alas, almost never allow consumers to regain normal functioning of their digestive tracts.

I was not satisfied with the idea of just taking a drug to fight against aerophagia, which I considered to be a mere symptom of a disturbance the cause of which I wanted to understand. As mainstream medicine could do nothing for me in what was considered to be a benign case, I simply had to fend for myself to understand why, all of a sudden, I seemed to be suffering from stomach acid and what I could do to cure it.

I have never believed in the quick fix of allopathic remedies. The respite that they give us must be paid for later on and sometimes at too high a price given the temporary comfort obtained. I believe that allopathic medicines are there to help us every now and then in times of crisis, but we need to figure out for ourselves why our bodies have become imbalanced and sick and what to do about it. We are all responsible for our health, and we first need to rely on ourselves to stay healthy. I believe that we are absolutely wrong when we imagine that we can neglect the most elementary rules of mental and physical hygiene and believe that a miracle quick-fix drug will give us back the well-being that we have lost due to our unhealthy lifestyles.

At the height of my crisis, I sometimes took the antacid prescribed by the doctor. I was intentionally limiting its use because of its many disastrous known side effects. When I could, I preferred to endure the attacks rather than taking the risk of paying dearly afterwards for the little comfort that an allopathic antacid could afford me. A little later, I started looking for alternatives to allopathic medicine, that is, ways to relieve myself free of side effects.

I then turned to acupuncture, which allowed me to relax, find a more peaceful sleep, and sometimes, but not always, alleviate my sudden bouts of aerophagia. After the acupuncture sessions, my stomach, which generally felt cold, regained its warmth. I felt energy circulating again in my solar plexus and I digested better, all with the only side effect of severely straining my budget, since weekly acupuncture was expensive and not covered by state healthcare. Acupuncture was a good replacement for antacid medication, but like allopathy it did not cure me. I decided after a few months to try my luck with homeopathy.

The homeopathic doctor recommended by a friend spent a whole hour speaking with me and asking me questions. It was very nice! He attributed my intestinal disturbances to stress, and he prescribed me several remedies at various dilutions to determine which would be the most effective. After many unsuccessful attempts, finally the combination of two homeopathic remedies worked very well and relieved me as well as allopathic medicine, without equaling the results I had achieved with acupuncture. Homeopathic remedies allowed me to space out the acupuncture sessions, so I continued chugging along for a few years with these homeopathic remedies and a monthly acupuncture session. I slept a little better and had fewer aerophagia crises that passed more quickly. But I had become overweight; my once slim waistline had become such a distant memory that it was barely believable. My skin had lost its freshness, I had large age spots on my cheeks, and many other problems, which I have listed below.

I felt I had entered a spiral of physical imbalances, sudden bouts of depression and weariness, and dependency on homeopathy and acupuncture. I felt that not one of the doctors I had consulted had found the cause of my suffering and understood what to do so that I could really heal. I was the one in my body and thus best placed to understand what was wrong with it, but I could not figure it out. I was determined to battle my way out of this sad state into which I was sinking deeper and deeper.

I wanted to understand why I had come to this while I had not changed my lifestyle. I continued somehow to do exercise, eat organic foods, and live as healthily as possible. Five years passed before I found the solution, five years in which my health steadily declined to the point that I decided to work from home so that I could rest when I needed it. Other annoyances had added to the aerophagia. I will list a few of them for you:

- Lumbar pain;
- Weight gain, especially on the stomach and waist, despite my eating sensibly and taking regular exercise;
- Circulatory problems, tensions in the legs, discomfort behind the knees, cold feet and hands;
- Frequent indigestion and vomiting;
- Nauseous states;
- Large age spots on my cheeks;
- Dry eyes;
- Burst blood vessels in the whites of the eyes;
- Tension behind the eyeballs and pain in the eyes;
- Blurred vision and reduced visual acuity;
- Tinnitus (ringing in the ears);
- Reduced perception of the taste of food;
- Yellowish color of the whites of the eyes;
- Nervousness;
- Insomnia or drowsiness;
- Loss of zest for life;
- Alternation between diarrhea and constipation;
- Joints pain, mainly in my hands;
- Chronic fatigue;
- Nightmares;
- Night sweats, especially on the upper body;
- Sudden feelings of coldness throughout the body before the onset of an aerophagia crisis;

- Increasingly bothersome premenstrual symptoms, with increasingly unbearable swelling and heaviness of the breasts, starting in the middle of the cycle and giving me very little respite;
- Phases of depression, low mood, and discouragement;
- Frequent colds.

I tried to do my best to live despite all these discomforts. I began to avoid as much as possible anything that could stress or depress me, since most of the doctors I had consulted attributed my symptoms to stress. To keep my spirits as high as possible and avoid a depression that would probably have made me dependent on antidepressant medication, I tried to keep negative people away, and I only read upbeat and constructive or humorous books. It was around this time that I decided to get rid of my television and stop reading the newspapers, because mainstream media is so full of depressing news that I realized I would be better off without it. We can endure it in small doses without repercussions when everything is going well in our lives, but when we are doing badly, we instead need news that cheers us up! I started looking for websites with jokes and funny videos. I dragged myself through each day as best I could. I also started working at home as a freelancer so that I could rest when needed and make myself comfortable during a crisis. At that time, I spent many hours looking for alternative remedies for treating all my little health issues, which were starting to snowball and undermine all my vitality.

During a trip to England, I read in a book of homeopathy that dry eyes are caused by age and that there was a homeopathic remedy to help. I tried it, but unfortunately it

10

didn't work for me. A doctor prescribed me eye baths, but on buying the bottle at the pharmacy, I noticed that it contained chemical preservatives. One of my friends had just had a severe allergy due to an allopathic eye wash, which made me opt for a more natural solution (and obviously one which was much more expensive and not covered by national healthcare). I didn't want to take the risk of putting such chemicals in my eyes, which were already in a sorry state. I found some natural blueberry floral water in an organic shop that did the job very well. Whenever I had to travel, I dreaded the dry air of airplanes and TGVs (French high-speed trains), and I carried my eye remedies wherever I went.

To tackle my poor eyesight and the unpleasant strain in my eyes, I took yoga classes, which gave me some relief. As for the yellowish color of the whites of my eyes, I thought it was also due to age and since it didn't hurt, it was the least of my worries. I was much more embarrassed by these huge age spots that had appeared on my face, mainly on my cheeks. Finally, I must say that I could no longer recognize myself in the mirror, physically or morally! People around me often told me that I had lost my zest for life and that it was strange that I was overweight with all the exercise I did and my healthy diet.

I did some research about how to remove age spots and I learned that I could depigment my skin with creams or even go to a cosmetic surgery clinic to have it done with laser therapy. Since these creams were expensive and not without their side effects, and the results were far from guaranteed, I didn't even bother trying them. I partially solved the problem by equipping myself with sun hats and sunscreens to protect my face, given that dermatologists claimed that sun was conducive to the onset of those ugly age spots.

To relieve my premenstrual symptoms, I consulted a homeopath who prescribed me hormones in homeopathic doses. I had endured these pains for several years, and I was so happy to find swift relief that I simply regretted not having consulted this doctor sooner. Unfortunately, it all started again after six months, and this time the homeopathic remedies did not work anymore. Therefore, I consulted a doctor who concluded that my premenstrual symptoms were caused by unresolved conflicts with my mother and also by stress and nervousness. He prescribed me remedies to calm me down, which I was in severe need of by that time.

Everything I took to deal with all the new symptoms that were bothering me was just a stopgap. Nothing restored my good health. Notwithstanding my healthy lifestyle, I had put on a lot of fat on my stomach, and the slender waist I had before my forties was but a distant memory. I was desperate and helpless in the face of my weight gain. Diets and exercise were fruitless. I had to resign myself to changing my wardrobe accordingly: no more pants, since I couldn't stand them anymore, and no more tight-fitting clothing in which I was uncomfortable and which no longer fit me. Over time, my attacks of aerophagia ceased to confine themselves to the night; instead, they could occur at any time, so I needed to wear loose clothing to be comfortable. Finally, I was so desperate that I even consulted a few healers, to no avail.

To understand what digestion is and how to improve it, I acquired several medical books on the digestive system, as well as books about diet explaining the bad food combinations which led to bloating. I also tried a number of herbal teas that didn't do much for me. Despite all this advice, herbal teas, and a strict diet, I could not alleviate these digestive troubles. As soon as I ate something, even a very light steamed dish, I felt like I had a stone in my stomach. It bore no resemblance to the normal feeling of contentment and well-being one should have after a good meal, eaten in the right conditions, when one is in good health.

Despite all these troubles, I continued exercising regularly and eating as well as possible. Sometimes I even stopped eating for a whole day and it gave me a lot of relief, which unfortunately was only temporary.

I forgot to mention charcoal, which was recommended by a friend and which I often used during these years. Charcoal helped me a lot. Activated vegetable charcoal is sold in pharmacies, often in the form of capsules or tablets full of sugar! Sugar is conducive to bloating, boxes of powdered sugar-free charcoal that can be purchased at organic food stores. Vegetable charcoal, which is considered a food supplement, is an adsorbent. It is of great interest in the case of bloating, since it eliminates gas and cleanses the intestine. Charcoal cannot be ingested if you take medication or birth control pills, because it cancels their effects. In health food stores, there are also combinations of clay and plants, or charcoal and plants that help remove gas. There are also all kinds of herbal teas for this purpose, and also essential oil blends. For my part, I tried all the natural remedies I could find.

Despite all I did, over the years my condition only got worse. I had become a shadow of myself, a fat shadow! I dragged myself around, tired and more and more uncomfortable in my body. My stomach had become for me like a ball and chain. All the books that I had read on digestion, all the mainstream or alternative doctors that I had consulted over the course of the years had not led me to understand why I had come to this and how I could regain good health.

As I started to lose faith and resign myself to a life lived in this state, like so many others, I was lucky to find at an organic fair, on the stand of a vendor of devices for sprouting seeds, a little book on intestinal hygiene written by a French doctor.

I had at home a whole collection of books by learned doctors, acupuncturists, naturopaths, hypnotists, homeopaths, healers, masseurs, etc. But I had never found in French bookstores one on intestinal hygiene. None of the many doctors consulted in the previous five years had ever even mentioned the subject! Curious, I bought this little book, which I read the same evening. Finally, fortune had smiled on me, and thanks to this book I finally understood the origin of all my health issues. It changed my life. Without this book, I don't think I would be here thirteen years later, still alive, rejuvenated, and in great shape to write this testimonial.

The author of the book claimed that to maintain a healthy digestive system, you just need to have good gut hygiene and that there are several very simple ways to cleanse the intestines, of which more later. It was simply the clogging of my colon that was interfering with the proper functioning of my body by poisoning it over time. All the symptoms that arise from poor intestinal hygiene can be treated by so many natural remedies or specific allopathic medicines with little result, because the underlying problem at the root of all these imbalances remains ignored. Instead, by cleansing the colon, all these symptoms disappear. Having good intestinal hygiene is really not complicated and is accessible to everyone. I will now tell you about my experiences with intestinal hygiene practices.

CHAPTER 1: WHAT COLON CLEANSING IS?

It is not my purpose to teach you the anatomy of the digestive system. Doctors excel in this field and yet, despite their science and sophisticated drugs, they fail to effectively relieve those afflicted by little digestive problems that, in the long run, snowball and ruin their health. They have the same "little problems," and many have never heard of intestinal hygiene as it is no longer taught in medical schools.

However, the book on intestinal hygiene that I found had been written by a doctor. He explains how the digestive system works, how the intestines gradually become clogged, and how to cleanse them with enemas and colon hydrotherapy. He gives examples of spectacular eliminations of waste obtained thanks to colonic irrigations. The cases cited are truly impressive. However, I have never seen such huge things come out of my intestines. A thin layer of compacted feces lining the walls of the colon is enough to disrupt the proper functioning of the entire body. Interestingly, his listing of all the health issues derived from a clogged colon perfectly matched all those I had experienced. Therefore, after reading his book, I decided to have colonic irrigations, despite my doctor claiming it was dangerous and useless because the colon naturally cleans itself.

I cannot reproduce excerpts from this book on intestinal hygiene because of copyright law. But, I found a public domain book, published in 1936 by Victor Pauchet, a

17

French doctor, entitled *Le chemin du Bonheur*, in which there is a very interesting passage on the issue.

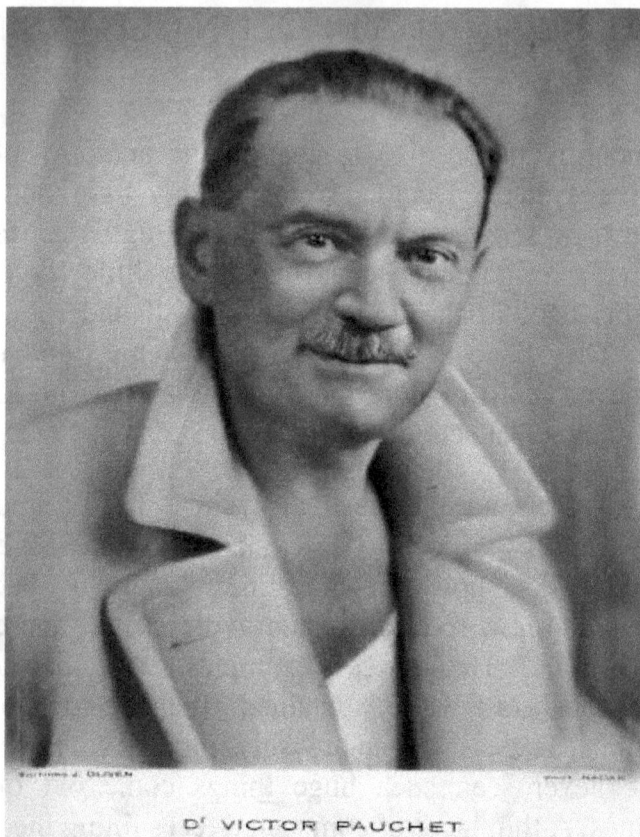

Dᴿ VICTOR PAUCHET

Devices for colonic irrigation did not exist in France at that time, so he does not mention this practice. However, his book is still relevant today because, through his medical experience, he proves how much a congested colon is harmful to health. Let us thank him here for his valuable testimonial. In his days, some doctors were seriously interested in the issue of constipation and were aware of its harmful effects on health. This is no longer the case today, as almost all of us believe that by taking laxatives this "minor health issue" will be easily solved.

Unfortunately, allopathic or natural laxatives taken for too long only make the situation worse over time by irritating the body.

After reading the book I found in the fair, I thought "Finally! I now understand the root of all my troubles. It is only because I have a clogged bowel!" And I wondered why none of the many doctors I had consulted prescribed having my colon cleansed. I soon realized that these unfortunate doctors were often sicker than me and did not even know how to heal themselves. Doctors suffer from bodily disorders that gradually set in when they lose colon cleanliness. They take it as something inevitable due to aging and put up with it as much as they can. They have never heard about intestinal hygiene in medical school, and most often it seems quite absurd to them to be able to heal (or avoid) many diseases just by cleaning the intestines.

One of them - having noticed my transformation and the exceptional improvement of my health - decided to have colonic irrigations, to his greatest benefit. He told me he really regretted never having been taught about this practice at medical school. Thanks to it, he could heal his long-lasting hypoglycemia.

CHAPTER 2: A FAMOUS FRENCH SURGEON'S OPINION ON THE DISASTROUS CONSEQUENCES OF CLOGGED COLON

This is a translation of some excerpts of Dr. Victor[1] Pauchet's book, *Le Chemin du Bonheur*, pages 51 to 59:

"What are the ailments and diseases caused by constipation on the right side of the colon? Constipation does not give trouble as long as it stays on the left side, but when it goes up to the right side of the colon, then the symptoms of intestinal poisoning appear. Here they are:

a) <u>Nervous disorders</u> - People with intestinal poisoning are tired and lifeless; some are lazy and depressed. In contrast, others are excited; some are drowsy, others suffer from insomnia and are unable to get good sleep without nightmares. Intellectual or physical effort is painful.

One should suspect constipation in the right side of the colon in people who complain of laziness, migraines, intercostal neuralgia, sciatica, facial pain, and breast pain. Blood laden with intestinal poisons permeates the nerves and interferes with the function of the nervous system.

Ten years ago a young man was sent to me with the diagnosis of a brain tumor; the pain in his head was

---

[1] Dr Victor Pauchet (1869-1936) ;
https://fr.wikipedia.org/wiki/Victor_Pauchet

excruciating and he requested trepanation at all costs. The X-ray of the colon showed constipation in the right side, which was the cause of his neuralgia. The patient was operated on for his constipation and his headaches disappeared.

Most people with intestinal poisoning are sad and unhappy; they get up tired, discouraged, and do not have a zest for life. Most young girls have no taste for marriage, and if they do get married they make sad wives, making their husbands miserable, either through their temper or their constant fatigue. Ladies, do not push your daughters into marriage as long as their intestines are poorly emptied; otherwise they will be unhappy and their husbands will leave them. They will complain of migraines, fatigue, slight fever, and will stay lying on a couch for two or three days a month, which will annoy the spouse tremendously. Fortunately, these young girls with a conservative gut don't have a great taste for marriage; it is the parents who push them in this direction. They are wrong.

All these chronically poisoned patients are cataloged as hysterical, nervous, neurasthenic, and neuropathic; the doctor and family often give the patient the responsibility for their miseries. "You can see that it's nervous" said a mother to her daughter. "You can see that you are not sick," said the annoyed husband to his discouraged wife. And yet, if the mothers had their daughters' digestive tracts X-rayed, the diagnosis would be made and the girl would be cured! The happiness of a family deserves an X-ray and a liter of paraffin.

b) Skin disorders - Chronically constipated people have dark skin, especially in the flexion folds of the limbs, at

22

the base of the neck, and on the back of the arms. The skin seems dirty, badly washed; their sweat is smelly. There is acne; hairs grow where they shouldn't and don't grow where they should. The hair falls out early and, on the other hand, an abundant down is seen on the cheeks, the forearms, and the backside of the arms, to such an extent that some women do not want to wear short sleeves. A large number of skin diseases like eczema and itching have no other causes. Body fat melts, limbs lose weight, body shapes and contours become angular; too loose skin wilts early, causing ugliness and premature old age.

c) Digestive disorders - Chronically constipated people do not have an appetite, nor do they enjoy life and action; their tongues are heavy, their breath foul, their mouths bad and bitter. All the 'appetizers' have no effect; digestion is slow and meals are heavy on the stomach. Doctors utter the words dyspepsia, chronic appendicitis, and enteritis, and dispatch these patients to spas, to no avail. They go to the bandager, who puts on a belt, then a ball, without improving the static of the belly.

d) Circulatory disorders - Chronically constipated people are chilly; their nose, ears, hands, and feet are cold. Frostbite is common. These so-called anemic or arthritic patients love hot weather, high altitudes, and do not like staying at the seaside or cold seasons. They often have heart palpitations and shortness of breath during brisk walking.

e) Muscle atrophy - The muscular system is weak; muscles soften and people love to lie down; they are round-shouldered and we see scoliosis appear in young girls, flat feet and *genu valgum* in boys. The ptosis or fall of the viscera obliges the patients to wear a corset or a belt.

f) Condition of the breasts - When a woman complains of pain or tumors of the breast, consider doing a fluoroscopy of the digestive tract. Most of the time, lesions in the breast are of intestinal origin. It suffices that the intestine empties regularly for the breast to become again normal. I have found that in women with breast cancer, eight out of ten times there is a delay in bowel movement. If they had been told about it ten or fifteen years before, they would never have had a breast tumor or cancer.

g) Glandular disorders - The poisons carried by the blood affect the glands and especially the breasts, the thyroid gland, the ovaries, all the endocrines, etc. Many women are forced to lie down for a few days or a few hours during each menstrual period. Many of them do not have children; others undergo surgery that does not improve their health.

h) Joint disorders - Often chronically constipated people are affected by joint pain, chronic rheumatism, and deformation of the joints. A large number of children treated in marine sanatoria for tuberculosis of the bones, glands, and joints have right-sided constipation, and if it had been cleared their infirmities would not have existed.

d) Respiratory failure - Intestinal poisoning suppresses the need and energy to breathe deeply. Poor breathing, in turn, affects the functioning of the bowel. Most people with intestinal poisoning have a pale or dark complexion, elongated face, narrow chest, hunched back, open mouth...

How do you recognize a subject with intestinal poisoning?

To recognize this common condition, you just need to think about it; to confirm this hypothesis it is necessary to: a) subject the person to X-rays; and b) perform a bacteriological examination of the stools. The number of undiagnosed chronically constipated people labeled with the most fanciful diagnoses is huge. They are treated for arthritis, neurasthenia, anemia, dyspepsia, enteritis, salpingitis, metritis, sterility, etc. The surgeons operate on them - without result - for mobile kidney, appendicitis, deviation of the matrix, and cystic ovaries. At orthopedists they are treated for a deformity of the spine and flat feet. Bandagers try all models of straps and belts on them. Dentists treat them for suppuration of the gums. Otorhinolaryngologists remove their tonsils and adenoids. Specialists in skin diseases treat itching, hair loss, excessive body hair, smelly sweat, and frostbite. Nervous system specialists treat them for neurasthenia, neuropathy, hysteria, etc.

You will find these misdiagnosed patients in all the spas; in Vichy, they take care of their liver and stomach; in Luxeuil of their ovarian disorders; in Châtel-Guyon and in Plombières of their enteritis and constipation; in Bourbon, the Archambault, and in Dax, of their pains and rheumatism; in Uriage, they treat diseases of the skin and throat; in Divonne-les-Bains, they take showers; in Evian and Vittel, they clean their kidneys; and at La Bourboule or at Mont-Dore, they attempt to disinfect their bronchi. In Switzerland they make the fortune of the diet houses. These 'poisoned' people thus run, all their lives, after health, try all the remedies and finally die of tuberculosis, arteriosclerosis, or cancer!

How do you know that all these dissatisfied with life carry in the gut the cause of their miseries? Through X-rays and bacteriological examination of the stools. But you might say, "I don't need an X-ray to know if I'm emptying my gut or not, as long as I'm regular." You are wrong; your regularity may be only apparent. Put a bucket under an open faucet; it will always be full, although the water is constantly overflowing. Only X-rays tell the truth and it takes four or five successive fluoroscopic examinations (one every twelve hours)."

This doctor was so convincing. He was one of the most famous French surgeons and the inventor of new tools and techniques for surgery of the digestive tract. He was enjoying vibrant health until his death in a car accident. He was 67 years old.

Let's now speak about modern colonic irrigation.

CHAPTER 3: THE UNFOLDING OF A COLONIC IRRIGATION SESSION

After reading the book on intestinal hygiene I bought at the fair, I immediately decided to have colonic irrigations despite the fact that I was afraid and believed it would be very unpleasant and painful.

I could not find the contact details of the author of the book and I searched for another colon therapist in Paris. There were very few of them at the time. I chose one who seemed peaceful and gentle. She was busy when I called her and offered to call me back. She did, and I took my time describing my case. She explained to me the unfolding of a colon irrigation session and what I had to eat the day before in order to prepare. I made an appointment with her for my first colonic irrigation, which took place at the end of November 2000. Yes, I had finally managed to figure out what to do to "deflate"!

Before the first session I had to prepare myself by ingesting flax seeds in the evening for a few days. Flax seeds can be purchased at organic food stores. Put a tablespoon of seeds in a cup with a little water. Let them soak for a few hours and drink it all (the seeds and the mucilage that has formed around it) at bedtime. This acts as a mild laxative, which starts cleansing the colon. The day before the colonic irrigation I had to eat only cooked vegetables and fruits. I could eat nothing just before the sessions. The naturopath advised me to wait a few hours after the colonic and then eat some boiled white rice. (Later on, during my travels, I saw that in other countries practitioners advised different methods for preparing for a colonic, and different foods just after it. In fact, it's up to each of us to find out what is best for us. There are also therapists who perform colonic irrigations without asking the patient to prepare for it.)

On the day of the appointment this experienced naturopath greeted me very kindly in her office first so she could explain the functioning of the colon, showing me a poster of the anatomy of the digestive system that was on the wall, and how the colonic irrigation session was going to unfold. She inspected my stomach and waist and declared that I would need to do three colonic irrigations, with a two weeks gap in-between because I was extremely congested. After that I would just need one irrigation in fall and another in spring to stay well.

On the office wall there was a large anatomy poster showing the digestive system. I looked at it with great curiosity because it was unlike anything I had seen before on the subject; it also showed the links between areas of the colon and areas of the body and organs. According to this chart, problems in the eyes are linked to congestion of an area in the *caecum*. The naturopath also asked me about my diet and lifestyle. She concluded that I was eating and living healthily. As she spoke, I thought that none of the many medical books I had read mentioned colon irrigation or intestinal hygiene. What a pity for all of us!

I then entered the treatment room, where the naturopath left me alone for a while to make myself comfortable. She gave me a warm pair of socks because feet often get cold during colon irrigation. She also gave me a napkin to preserve my intimacy. Once I was ready, she walked into the treatment room and explained how the hydrotherapy device worked. I have photographed it and you can see it below.

Picture of a colon hydrotherapy machine:

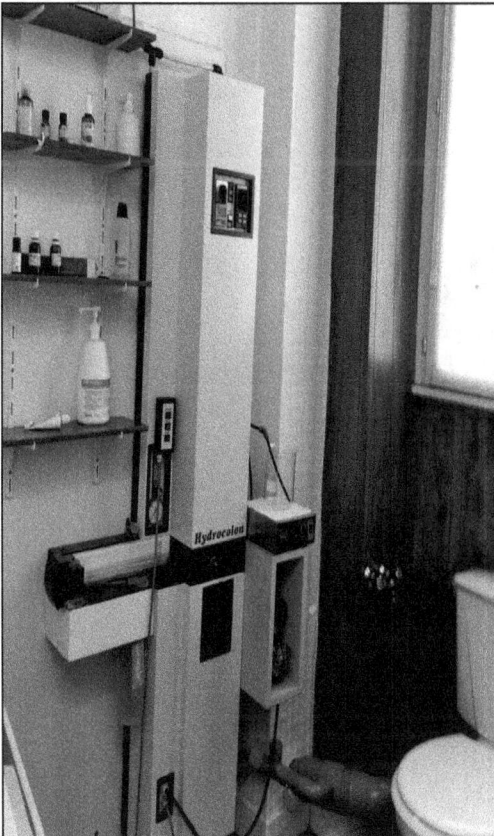

She took out of a sealed package a cannula and pipe. Then she attached the cannula to the pipe and connected the pipe to the hydrotherapy machine. She told me that the pipe and cannula are disposable, and are thrown away after the session. At the tip of the cannula are two holes.

One of them is for injecting water, the other is for sucking up water with the feces it has detached.

Picture of the cannula and pipe:

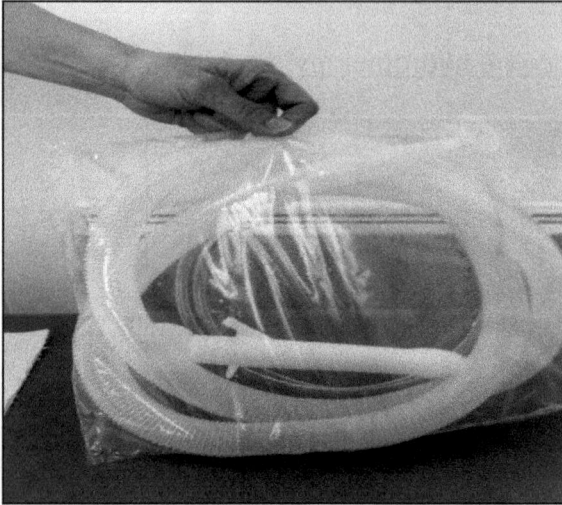

On the machine the therapist can regulate the temperature and pressure of the water. The system varies according to the different devices used. About ten centimeters of the piping that goes through the machine is transparent and illuminated, allowing the therapist (and the patient, if she wishes) to have a look at what is being eliminated during the session. This way the therapist can better advise patients accordingly about their diet mistakes. Indeed, this allows detection of them. For example, eating a lot of dairy products may result in expelling large amounts of mucus during colon hydrotherapy. I turned on my left side and she gently inserted the cannula into my rectum after lubricating it. Once the cannula was inserted, I got onto my back again and the irrigation session began. It lasted about an hour, during which the therapist massaged my stomach to help detach the old waste. The most unpleasant moment was the introduction of the cannula; the rest of the session was a really enjoyable belly massage, laughter, and chatter. As soon as I sensed some pressure, the machine automatically stopped injecting water. (This is not the case with all machines, some naturopaths have less sophisticated devices requiring manual intervention in case of pressure.)

After the first session, I felt free from the heavy weight I had carried in my stomach for all these years: what a joy! But it wasn't until the third session that my body released a lot of old stuff. After three sessions, I lost my stomach fat, regained a much slimmer waist, and lost some weight. My complexion became fresh and rosy again; the once-yellowish whites of my eyes were bluish-white again, and the two large "age" spots on my face had almost completely disappeared. I no longer had back pain, no more tension and heaviness in my legs, no more circulatory problems, no more nightmares, almost no more bloating, no more digestive problems, no more dry eyes, no more red eyes, no more pain and tension behind the eyeball. My sleep became peaceful, and I regained my natural zest for life and my good humor.

A week after the third session the naturopath called to ask how I was doing. I was well, but I couldn't resist playing a joke on her. I told her that despite the three colon irrigations, I still had a big problem. Surprised, she was curious to know what it was. I told her that for the past five years I had spent my life farting and seeking how to heal all my many health issues, and now I had no idea what I could do to keep busy! It triggered laughter on the other end of the line!

31

These three sessions had produced such a spectacular and visible improvement in my appearance and in my health that it struck a number of people around me; they asked if I was returning from vacation, if I had changed my diet, or performed cosmetic surgery on my stomach and waist. Some friends were puzzled by my sudden rejuvenation and asked me how I had achieved it. Everyone, men and women, were amazed at this radical positive change.

At the time, I was too shy to share this experience with people other than some of my closest friends who were open enough to listen to me. Among my close friends to whom I spoke about my colonic irrigations, several decided to have colonic irrigations, too. A friend of mine who had been overweight for years and used to wear only loose clothing was transformed after having three colonic irrigations. I saw her for the first time, elegant and wearing a skirt! Sadly, however, she did not develop a good diet and lifestyle habits and ended up losing the benefit of her irrigations after a while. Colonic irrigations do help maintain a good figure and health, but a healthy physical and emotional lifestyle is necessary to avoid clogging the digestive tract again and again.

As far as I am concerned, during the five years of health disorders I had removed stimulants (coffee, tea, alcoholic drinks), overly fatty dishes, canned goods, frozen foods, bad food combinations, and then meat and dairy products. I had started to feed myself just like the yogis of India! In addition, since I had continued regularly going to the gym despite all my embarrassments, once I was cleansed by the colonic irrigations my body did not take long in returning naturally to better health and staying that way.

As a result, the benefits of irrigation lasted much longer for me than for the friend I told you about. But that did not mean I regained perfect health. I was still fragile and easily disturbed. At times I still had a little bloating and some small crises of aerophagia. I sometimes suffered from slow transit. But these little problems accounted for just about 5% of all the troubles I had endured before the colonic irrigations and were therefore a lot easier to manage. Whenever I started feeling a bit constipated, I would do an enema, take flax seeds for a few days, and eat more steamed vegetables that contained lot of water. I was usually well during the two or three months after a colonic irrigation. After that, I had to consider another session.

I am now going to speak about the utility of enemas. Alas! None of the many doctors I consulted in my life regarding constipation problems ever advised me to use one. Instead, they prescribed laxatives, which have side effects and make the bowels lazier and lazier. Enemas are inexpensive, provide quick relief, do not render the bowels lazy, and have no side effects. You can buy an enema bucket, a bulb syringe, an enema bag, or an enema kit, at the pharmacy or online.

The enema bucket which can easily be ordered from pharmacies and costs just under $20, is a rigid plastic container that can hold two liters of water. It is sold with a pipe of about one meter, at the end of which there is a cannula and a tap (two cannulas are often supplied with the pitcher, one rectal and the other vaginal).

Picture of an enema bucket:

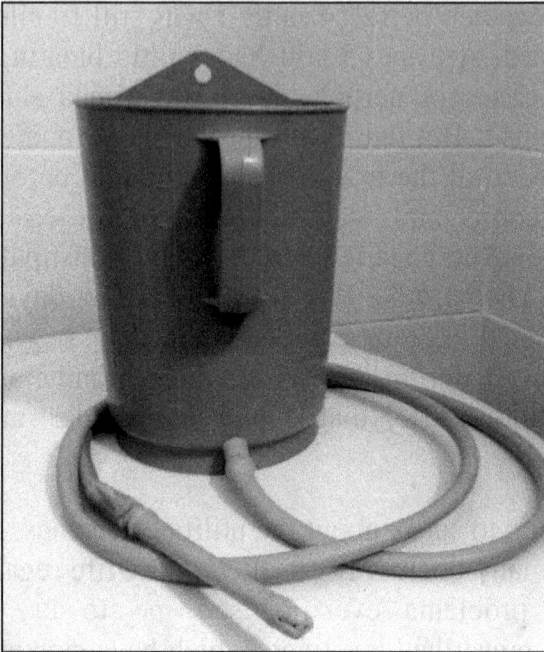

All you have to do is boil some water, let it cool down, put it in the container, lubricate the cannula, and insert it into the rectum while you are comfortably lying either on your back or on your right side, or other positions you prefer. Then let the water flow from the container into the colon. After some time, the intestines will empty by reflex.

Some people add salt to the water to prevent spasms. (Even without salt, I never had spasms doing enemas.) Others use infusions of chamomile or other plants. Some use laxatives this way, unfortunately having the same side effect as ingested laxatives. Allopathic or natural laxatives are supposed to allow a deep cleansing of the intestines, but this is not true. I have tried almost everything, even the trendy magnesium chloride! They all cause a call for water inside the intestines, diarrhea, and severe disturbances without effectively clearing the colon. Beware of advertisements for miraculous enema cures, which are in fact laxatives taken rectally instead of the usual oral route. They are expensive and have the same drawbacks as other laxatives. Beware also of advertisements about colon cleansing products that show ugly big clumps that have come out of the intestines after ingesting these miracle cures. In fact, what comes out is just the advertised products themselves, transformed by moisture and heat inside the body. You can get the same result by mixing these products with water and keeping the mixture warm for a while. By the way, on *YouTube* you can see videos that advertise these products and others that expose the truth about them.

With a pitcher you let in two liters of water while massaging your stomach. This enema can be done in the privacy of your home and will help you maintain good intestinal hygiene whenever you need it. It's easy to do, free, and doesn't have the drawbacks of laxatives. In my opinion, laxatives should be used only exceptionally and they should be mild. Many other non-invasive solutions are available when we need help to empty the intestines.

Colon irrigation, which uses a much larger amount of water, is much more effective than a two liters enema. It will help cleanse the whole colon. By experimenting with both, you will see the difference between a home enema and colon therapy. As a comparison, an American author claims that it takes a dozen enemas to achieve the same result as one colonic. For my part, I have observed that even a dozen enemas do not give the results of good colon irrigation. During colonic irrigation, water circulates in large quantities throughout the colon while it is being massaged. This makes it much more likely for the patient to clear up the stagnant waste from the intestinal wall. It is important to choose a therapist with whom you feel comfortable and relaxed. It will ease everything and the bowels will be more prone to release the old waste. There is also a psychological dimension to colon cleansing: the more we are ready to let go, the better results we can achieve.

The advantage an enema has over colonic irrigation is that it can be done at home and is much less tiring. As far as I am concerned, fatigue for one or two days is the only drawback to colon therapy. I have also noticed that it works better when the weather is not cold. Although some people tolerate irrigations without much fatigue, after irrigation I sleep a lot. My face is tired and I tend to have dark circles around my eyes for a few days. I need an acupuncture session to restore the flow of energy in the solar plexus. Without an acupuncture session, my stomach stays cold for a few days because the energy flow is disturbed in this area. Therefore, it's only after a few days of rest and after an acupuncture session that I feel purified and in great physical shape again after a colonic irrigation. Most people are not that sensitive and can resume working and eating as usual after a colonic. It depends on each person.

You can use a foldable enema bag that is more practical for traveling than a pitcher. Some are disposable and you can easily find them on the internet or at pharmacies.

Picture of a foldable enema bag:

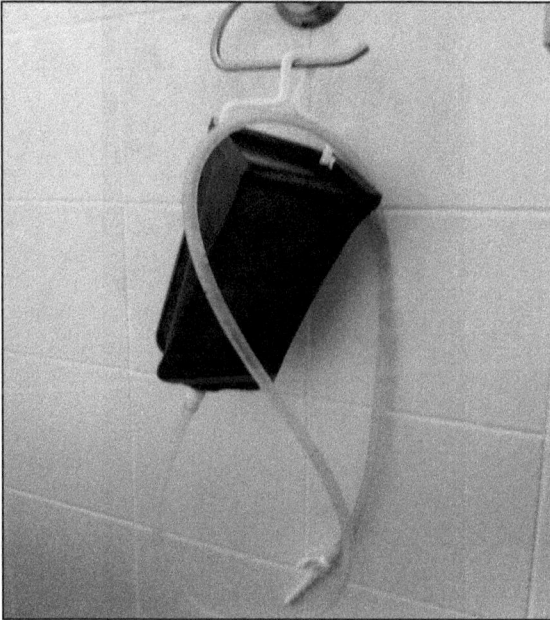

Enema bulbs syringes can also help when traveling. They are one of the least effective methods, due to the small amount of water used, but in some circumstances are much better than nothing.

Picture of an enema bulb:

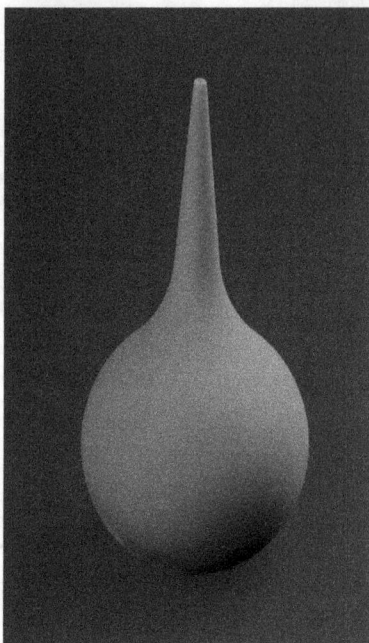

I was so happy with the results I achieved with my first three sessions of colon hydrotherapy that I continued with the same experienced and gentle practitioner. I had some colonics with other therapists during my travels, or when my therapist was not available. For ten years, I continued to have a colonic irrigation in spring and autumn, which I greatly needed each time because the tension in the legs, my nervousness, my fatigue, and my insomnia tended to recur, even though it was much milder than before my initial three sessions.

Two colonic irrigations a year kept me happy and healthy. It takes around 150 USD per session, much less than all I spent before in attempting to heal all the many symptoms deriving from my gut being clogged with waste. I hope that in the future health insurance will help cover preventive care costs instead of spending so much on disease. A lot of misery and suffering could be avoided this way, but of course it would not be to the taste of Big Pharma.

Years passed, and in October 2009 I did my usual fall colonic irrigation, which went very well. But for about a year, despite the irrigations, I felt that I needed to cleanse my body better. I thought that maybe I was congested in a higher part of the digestive tract and for this reason colon cleansing was not enough.

Therefore, I decided to fast for three days. It was a good idea, and I will tell you why.

CHAPTER 4: FASTING: A VERY EFFECTIVE MEANS FOR CLEANING THE DIGESTIVE TRACT

I did not eat at all the day before the colonic irrigation, nor the day after it as I had slept for a very long time. I then decided to continue fasting, drinking only herbal teas. Then I gradually added organic juices that I made at home with a juicer, mainly with carrots, beetroot, and grapes.

The beginning of the fast was a bit taxing; I felt weak because I had just had a colonic irrigation and had not yet visited my acupuncturist. After that, contrary to what I expected, all became easy and I even skipped the acupuncture session. I became filled by such a great peace and it seemed that a veil had been lifted from my eyes. I could see better and I felt better; I was much lighter and quieter. I thought that it was probably due to a cleansing of my liver and purification of my blood.

I was very surprised on the third day when I evacuated a lot of waste while I had eaten nothing for a while. By examining what I had eliminated, I realized that despite all the colonic irrigations done for the past nine years, and all I had done to clean my digestive tract, some part of my intestines seemed still lined with waste so dried out that it did not smell or look like feces, but rather looked like an amber-colored plastic mold of my colon.

My conclusion was that all the colon irrigations had relieved me a lot, but not completely cleansed my intestines. In fact, they cannot be as effective as a fast when the colon is cluttered with old, hard, and compacted material accumulated year after year. The one-hour duration of colonic irrigation is not enough to rehydrate and remove these old materials that are compacted, dried up, and attached to the intestinal walls for so long. An American author recommends having at least twelve colon irrigations over a short period of time and drinking lots of vegetable juices to effectively cleanse the colon.[2]

The intestines are alive and sensitive; they are not a mere pipe that you just have to unclog with water or other means. It is not easy to achieve gut cleanliness when, like me, you have waited too long and your intestinal walls are covered with a tight layer of compacted and dried waste. It takes a lot of patience, persistence, and determination. We have a second brain in our belly, an emotional brain. Fasting, by the calmness it induces, promotes relaxation, and relaxation is conducive to the intestines letting go of old stuff. When we fast under the right conditions, it is the body and not just the mind that decides to free itself from the past.

Finally, I fasted for seven days, and each day I eliminated some more very old, very hard and dried out feces, which looked like stones or molds of my intestinal walls. Then I gradually resumed a normal diet. Despite resuming a normal diet, my body continued for about a month to free itself from old matters that had clogged my bowels probably since my childhood.

---

[2] *Colon Health, The Key to a Vibrant Life*, Dr. Norman W. Walker

Now I still have colonic irrigations from time to time when I am not in the condition for fasting, or as a complement to fasting. Whenever I have a colonic, I fast the day before, the day of the colonic irrigation, and the day after. It is very efficient. Thanks to these combined practices of fasting and colonic irrigations, I have now regained great vitality and can happily participate in family celebrations and go to a restaurant with friends from time to time without worrying about my health. Quite simply, I live normally and in good health! Too bad I did not hear of colon cleansing earlier!

Finally, fasting is much more effective than anything else at clearing our bowels and purifying our bodies and minds. And it's free! But, it's not easy, and when it cannot be done, colonic irrigation is the best alternative to help cleanse the colon and stay healthy.

Here is the opinion of Dr. Victor Pauchet on fasting, taken from his book (pp. 17 and 18)

"FAST - Fasting is the best detoxification process that exists.

Fasting is about depriving yourself of food for twenty-four hours, forty-eight hours, or more. In this way, toxins are eliminated; the digestive tract rests; the vascular system is no longer tired with the addition of new amounts of nutrients. Anyone with an acute sickness must fast. Fasting should precede the treatment of most chronic diseases. Whenever you experience any discomfort you should put yourself on an absolute diet so that the body can rest. Personally, I have a lot of experience with fasting, because I recommend it to all my future patients. Most of them fast from two to eight days; obese people live exclusively on water or oranges for four, six, or eight weeks before surgery. During the fast, it is necessary to drink warm, slightly sweetened herbal teas: prune herbal tea, apple tea, herbal broth, etc. Hot drinks can be easily replaced with good quality, raw, juicy fruit, as long as they are perfectly chewed. The fast does not always need to be so strict; it may simply consist of skipping one or two meals per twenty-four hours. As a rule, NEVER EAT IF YOU ARE NOT HUNGRY."

CONCLUSION

When I was suffering from bloating, I often regretted that the body was so poorly devised by Mother Nature! But when I began fasting I changed my mind and thanked my body for sounding the alarm bells with all this bloating and discomfort. Without it, I would never have found that my bowels were congested, as I had regular bowel movements during all those years. Like almost everyone, I would have attributed all my little ailments to ageing and tried eliminating my symptoms with medication. And maybe I would have died from colorectal cancer, like so many people in modern civilized countries who have never heard about colon cleansing.

I might also have continued unnecessarily strict diets and ineffective sit-ups in the gym to flatten my stomach! When I think about people with clogged bowels having cosmetic surgery to flatten their stomachs by tightening the abdominal muscles and skin and removing their belly fat, I realize that I was very lucky to find a more natural path for recovering my good health and flat stomach.

The body is smart; it often informs us through our dreams about its condition. During all these years, I had recurring dreams about pants that were too tight, clogged toilets and sinks, problems with going to the bathroom because either there was no toilet or there were a lot of people waiting in the line for the toilet. I also dreamed about broken toilets and overflowing sinks and tubs. Another recurring theme in my dreams was related to the overgrowth of insects in my home. At this time I did not understand the meaning of these dreams. If I had, these dreams would have helped me a lot and saved me lots of suffering. In her interesting book *Your Dreams Can Save Your Health*, Anna Mancini gives other examples of common dreams alerting the dreamer that their body is poorly eliminating its waste. She also demonstrates that our body regularly informs us about its condition through our dreams. Let us listen to our bodies' messages and give them what they really need: love, care, healthy food, fresh air, a peaceful state of mind, and inner and outer cleanliness.

Good energy flow in the solar plexus is of prime importance to digest and eliminate well and stay healthy. When this flow is disturbed, the belly is cold instead of warm. Bad news, worries, or a dip in a pool with water that is too cold can disturb this flow of energy. When I have a big shock jamming my solar plexus, I stop eating and I visit an acupuncturist to restore the flow of energy if I am not able to do it on my own. Doctor Bach's rescue remedy also helps me a lot in this case.

Stress and negative feelings are conducive to poor digestion and elimination contributing to digestive tract clogs. This in turn increases stress, negativity, discouragement, fatigue, and low mood. It's a vicious circle. Prevention through fasting, enemas, and relaxation is what we should all do when we are still in a good condition.

Good health is priceless! Clearing my bowels made a huge difference in my life. I woke up refreshed and joyful instead of tired, and regained my energy and zest for life. I became more active and creative. My mind was clear again. Clogged intestines bog down the mind and we get a feeling of being hampered and heavy. We become slow, unmotivated, and kind of lazy.

I hope that this book convinced you about the importance of keeping the digestive tract clean to stay healthy and to live better and longer in a clean, healthy, radiant, and comfortable body.

I wish you all the best!

BIBLIOGRAPHY

Colon Health, The Key to a Vibrant Life, Dr. Norman W. Walker's

Your Dreams Can Save Your Life: How and Why Your Dreams Warn You of Every Danger: Tidal Waves, Tornadoes, Storms, Landslides, Plane Crashes, Assaults, Attacks, Burglaries, Etc, Anna Mancini

Your Dreams Can Save Your Health: Signs of Infectious Diseases in Dreams, Dreaming the Right Remedies, Accurate Diagnosis, and Early Detection of Diseases, Anna Mancini

Home Medicine Guide, Edgar Cayce

The Cure for All Diseases, Hulda Clark

The Curious Man, the life and works of Dr. Hans Nieper

The New Science of Healing, Louis Khune

Forbidden Health: Incurable Was Yesterday, Andreas Ludwig Kalcker

Mucusless Diet Healing System: Scientific Method of Eating Your Way to Health, Arnold Ehret

MMS Health Manual, Jim Humble

49

Écosystème intestinal & Santé optimale, Docteur G. MOUTON

Hygiène intestinale: Retrouvez la santé avec un côlon dépollué, Dr. Christian Tal Schaller

La Santé par l'hygiène intestinale, Dr. Monnier

Les 5 clés de la revitalisation de l'organisme, Désiré Mérien

Saintes Pilules, Petites histoires Satiriques et Humoristiques à Propos de nos Croyances Scientifiques et Médicales, Eva Lavie

OTHER BOOKS IN ENGLISH
BY LAURE GOLDBRIGHT

Menopause Free of Suffering: A Testimonial

Menopause is Not a Disease! Hot flashes, Low Mood, Weight gains, and Other Menopausal Symptoms Can Be Avoided

Summary:

The women in my family have always had a lot of symptoms before, during, and after menopause. I didn't want to suffer like them and I decided to react. I questioned our Western beliefs about menopause and did some research to find out how I could avoid the usual menopause ailments. I was determined to have a happy menopause, without hot flashes, mood swings, insomnia, nervousness, depression, cellulite buildup, age spots on the face, and accelerated aging. And I achieved it!

I realized that almost all the symptoms culturally attributed to menopause are actually due to other causes, which can be eliminated.

In this book, I will explain how I performed my investigation; then I will share some important information so that you, too, can avoid the hardships our culture usually condemns women to with the outbreak of menopause. Even if you are already suffering from some so-called "menopausal symptoms," it's not too late to take action to live a happy and healthy menopause. This little book is easy to read, free of medical jargon, and considers the spiritual dimension of women.

OTHER BOOKS
BY LAURE GOLDBRIGHT

Menopause Free of Suffering: A Testimonial

Vegetarian and Organic Paris

Gare à Vous les Virus !

Les Parisiens au Boulot, LOL !

10 Ans d'Études, 20 Ans de Chômage, C'est Ça la Vraie France

Bienvenue à Tous Au Concours Du Centre National de la Recherche Scientifique

CONTENTS

www.ingramcontent.com/pod-product-compliance
Lightning Source LLC
Chambersburg PA
CBHW060643280326
41933CB00012B/2139